# HEART ATTACK UNMASKED

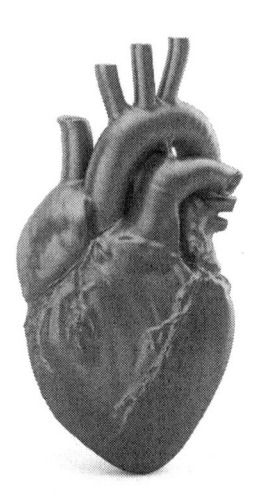

Defeating the Silent Assassin, Understanding Causes, and Healing for Life.

Cherie flores

## Copyright © 2023 By Cherie Flores

All rights reserved. No part of this publication may be reproduced, distributed, or transmitted in any form or by any means, including photocopying, recording, or other electronic or mechanical methods, without the prior written permission of the author, except in the case of brief quotations embodied in critical reviews and certain other noncommercial uses permitted by copyright law.

## TABLE OF CONTENT

**Chapter 1**

What is a Heart Attack?

Defining the Enemy

Types of Heart Attacks

How Heart Attacks Happen

**Chapter 2**

Risk Factors/causes of heart attack

Identifying the Culprits

Genetics and Family History

Lifestyle Choices

Age and Gender

## Chapter 3
Warning Signs and Symptoms
Listening to Your Body
Common Symptoms
Unusual Symptoms
When to Seek Help

## Chapter 4
Diagnosis and Medical Evaluation
Doctor's Visit
Diagnostic Tests
-Assessing Your Heart's Health

## Chapter 5
Understanding the Causes
Atherosclerosis: The Silent Buildup
High Blood Pressure
Cholesterol and Triglycerides
Diabetes and Insulin Resistance

## Chapter 6

Prevention Strategies

Diet and Nutrition (food to be eaten and avoided)

Exercise and Physical Activity

Stress Management

Medications and Treatments

## Chapter 7

Treatment Options

Medications

Angioplasty and Stenting

Bypass Surgery

Cardiac Rehabilitation

What to do when heart attack happens

Reversing Heart Attack

## Chapter 8

Life After a Heart Attack

Coping with the Aftermath

Lifestyle Changes for Recovery

Emotional Well-being

Support Systems

## Chapter 9

Healing and Recovery

Physical Rehabilitation

Cardiac Rehabilitation Programs

Diet and Exercise Plans   Monitoring Your progress.

# Chapter 1

## i. What is a Heart Attack?

A respiratory failure, medicinally known as myocardial dead tissue, happens when the blood supply to a piece of the heart muscle is impeded or diminished, for the most part because of the development of cholesterol and different substances (plaque) in the coronary veins. This can harm or annihilate a piece of the heart muscle, prompting different side effects and difficulties.

## 2. CHARACTERIZING THE ENEMY

The foe in this setting is atherosclerosis, a condition where plaque collects in the veins over the long haul, limiting them and possibly causing blockages. These plaques can burst, prompting the development of blood clusters, which can set off a cardiovascular failure by hindering blood stream to the heart.

## 3. TYPES OF HEART ATTACKS:

### I. ST-Portion Height Myocardial Localized necrosis (STEMI)

1: STEMI is a serious kind of cardiovascular failure.

2: It happens when there is a finished blockage of one of the coronary corridors, which supply blood to an enormous piece of the heart muscle.

**3**: Side effects are frequently serious and quick, including extreme chest torment, windedness, and different indications of pain.

**4:,** Quick clinical intercession is pivotal, normally including systems like angioplasty and stent situation to open the obstructed vein.

## ii Non-ST-Portion Height Myocardial Localized necrosis (NSTEMI)

**1:** NSTEMI is a less serious kind of cardiovascular failure contrasted with STEMI.

**2:** It happens when there is a halfway blockage or diminished blood move through a coronary course.

**3:** Side effects might be less extreme and can incorporate chest distress, weakness, and windedness.

**4:** Treatment for the most part includes drugs and analytic tests to survey the degree of the blockage.

## 4. How Coronary failures Happen:

### i:PLAQUE FORMATION

Respiratory failures frequently result from atherosclerosis, where greasy stores aggregate in the coronary corridors, limiting them.

### ii:PLAQUE RUPTURE

Plaque can crack or tear open, presenting its items to the circulation system.

### iii:Blood Clump Formation

The body's reaction to the cracked plaque can prompt the development of a blood coagulation at the site.

### iv:Hindered Artery

Assuming the blood coagulation is adequately enormous, it can impede the supply route, decreasing or totally removing blood stream to the heart.

### ii: Heart Muscle Damage

Without sufficient blood supply, the heart muscle begins to endure harm, and in the event that left untreated, this can prompt a coronary failure.

# Chapter 2

## 1. Risk Factors

Risk factors are conditions or ways of behaving that improve the probability of creating coronary illness or encountering a cardiovascular failure.

Distinguishing and dealing with these gamble factors is fundamental for keeping up with heart wellbeing and forestalling heart-related issues.

A cardiovascular failure, otherwise called a myocardial dead tissue, happens when there is a blockage in at least one of the coronary corridors, which supply blood to the heart muscle. This blockage is regularly brought about by the development of greasy stores (atherosclerosis) inside the supply routes. Here are the essential drivers and hazard factors for coronary episodes:

1. **Atherosclerosis**: This is the most well-known reason for coronary failures. Atherosclerosis is the continuous development of plaque (made out of cholesterol, fat, calcium, and different substances) on the inward walls of coronary supply routes. Over the long haul, this limits the corridors and confines blood stream to the heart.

2. **Coronary Corridor Illness (CAD)**: computer aided design alludes to the restricting or blockage of coronary courses because of atherosclerosis. It decreases the heart's oxygen supply, making it powerless against a respiratory failure.

**3. Blood Clots**: At times, a blood coagulation can frame on the outer layer of a plaque inside a coronary conduit. On the off chance that the coagulation turns out to be sufficiently enormous, it can totally obstruct blood course through the conduit, prompting a coronary failure.

**4. Spasm of Coronary Arteries**: now and again, the coronary veins can fit or tighten, decreasing blood stream to the heart. This can happen in people regardless of huge atherosclerosis.

**5. Risk Elements**:

Hypertension: Uncontrolled hypertension builds the burden on the heart and can harm courses.

**Elevated Cholesterol Levels**: Raised degrees of LDL (low-thickness lipoprotein) cholesterol, frequently alluded to as "awful" cholesterol, can prompt plaque development.

**Smoking**: Smoking harms the veins, diminishes oxygen supply, and adds to atherosclerosis.

**Diabetes**: Uncontrolled diabetes can harm veins and increment the gamble of atherosclerosis.

**Corpulence**: Overabundance weight can prompt circumstances like hypertension and diabetes, which are risk factors for coronary failures.

**Family Ancestry**: A family background of coronary illness can build your gamble.

Age and Orientation: The gamble of cardiovascular failure increments with age, and men are by and large at higher gamble than premenopausal ladies.

Actual Idleness: Absence of activity can add to heftiness and other gamble factors.

Stress: Constant pressure can influence the heart and lead to unfortunate adapting ways of behaving like indulging or smoking.

It means a lot to take note of that while these are the essential drivers and chance variables, cardiovascular failures can likewise happen because of more uncommon causes, for example, illicit drug use, certain prescriptions, extreme contaminations, or a tear in a coronary course (coronary corridor analyzation). Brief clinical consideration is significant in the event that you experience side effects of a coronary episode, for example, chest torment, windedness, or distress in the arms, back, neck, or jaw.

## 2. Distinguishing the Culprits

To distinguish the offenders behind coronary illness, it's vital to perceive and address the accompanying risk factors:

## 3. Hereditary qualities and Family History

Family ancestry assumes a critical part in coronary illness risk.

If direct relations, similar to guardians or kin, have a background marked by coronary illness, your gamble might be higher.

Hereditary elements can likewise add to coronary illness risk, yet way of life decisions stay significant in dealing with this gamble.

## 4. Way of life Choices

Way of life decisions are among the most powerful calculates heart wellbeing.

Undesirable propensities like smoking, an eating regimen high in immersed fats and handled food sources, absence of actual work, and unreasonable liquor utilization can fundamentally increment coronary illness risk.

Embracing a heart-solid way of life, which incorporates a fair eating routine, ordinary activity, and abstaining from smoking, can bring down these dangers.

## 5. Age and Gender

Age is a non-modifiable gamble factor; as we progress in years, the gamble of coronary illness increments.

Men are for the most part at higher gamble for coronary illness contrasted with ladies, yet the gamble for ladies increments after menopause.

Be that as it may, coronary illness can influence individuals of any age and sexual orientations, so zeroing in on counteraction and endanger the board over the course of life is significant.

HEART ATTACK UNMASKED

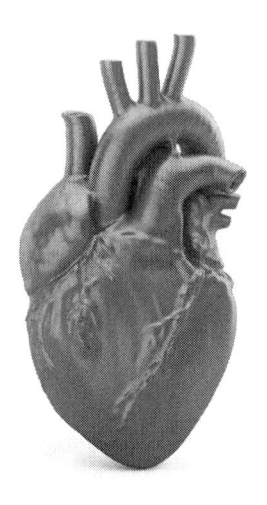

# CHAPTER 3

## 1. Signs and Side effects

Perceiving the signs and side effects of heart-related issues is critical for early mediation and looking for proper clinical assistance.

Heart-related side effects can shift from one individual to another, and some can be unobtrusive or unforeseen.

## 2. Paying attention to Your Body

Focusing on your body is fundamental with regards to heart wellbeing.

Assuming that you experience any uncommon or tenacious side effects, it's significant not to disregard them and to quickly look for clinical assessment.

## 3. Normal Side effects

**Normal heart-related side effects include**

i: Chest Agony or Inconvenience Frequently portrayed as a crushing, tension, or copying sensation.    ii: Shortness of Breath Trouble breathing or a sensation of windedness.

iii: Pain or Uneasiness in the Arms, Neck, Jaw, Back, or Stomach
Some of the time, heart-related agony can transmit to these areas.

**iv:** Fatigue, Surprising sluggishness or shortcoming.

**V:** Dizziness or Wooziness Feeling weak or shaky. **Vi:** Nausea or RegurgitatingvCertain individuals might encounter sickness or spewing as a side effect.

## Uncommon Side effects

While the above side effects are normal, it's critical to take note of that heart-related side effects can likewise be abnormal or uncommon.

These can incorporate side effects like virus sweats, torment in the upper back or between the shoulder bones, and distress that looks like acid reflux.

## When to Look for Help

**I:** It's vital to look for clinical assistance expeditiously assuming you experience any signs or side effects that you suspect might be connected with your heart.

**ii :** Don't defer in the event that you're uncertain; it's smarter to get really taken a look at by a medical services proficient to preclude any difficult issues.

**iii:** In the event that you or somebody you're with encounters abrupt and serious chest torment, windedness, or loss of awareness, call crisis benefits right away.

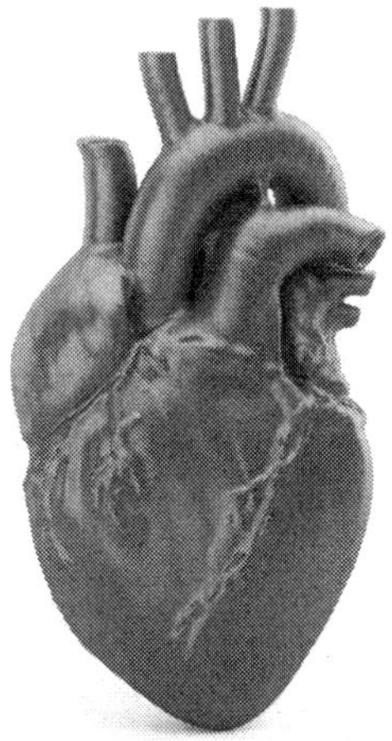

# CHAPTER 4

### Analysis and Clinical Evaluation

Diagnosing a coronary episode includes an exhaustive clinical assessment by medical services experts.

Expeditious and exact determination is critical to start the fitting treatment and limit heart muscle harm.

### Specialist's Visit

In the event that you suspect you're having a coronary failure or are encountering side effects, for example, chest torment or uneasiness, looking for sure fire clinical attention is fundamental.

Visiting the specialist or going to the trauma center is the most important phase in the demonstrative cycle.

## 3. Analytic Tests

- A few indicative tests might be performed to evaluate your heart's wellbeing and affirm the presence of a coronary failure:

### a. Electrocardiogram (ECG or EKG)

This test records the electrical action of your heart. It can uncover anomalies in your heart's musicality and recognize indications of a coronary episode.

### b. Blood Tests

Blood tests are taken to quantify heart biomarkers like troponin and creatine kinase-MB (CK-MB). Raised levels of these markers can show heart muscle harm.

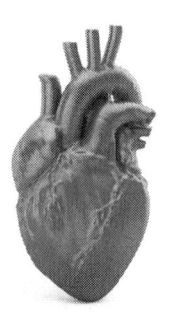

### c. Coronary Angiography

This methodology includes infusing a differentiation color into your coronary supply routes and taking X-beam pictures (angiograms) to distinguish blockages or limited courses.

### d. Echocardiogram

This ultrasound test makes pictures of your heart to survey its design and capability, deciding the degree of heart harm.

### e. Cardiac CT or MRI

These imaging strategies give nitty gritty photos of your heart and veins and can be utilized to assess heart construction and blood stream.

## 4. Surveying Your Heart's Health

In light of the consequences of these demonstrative tests, medical care experts can decide the area and seriousness of the respiratory failure.

Treatment choices, like drug, angioplasty, or sidestep a medical procedure, are then picked in view of the evaluation of your heart's wellbeing.

Early determination and mediation are basic in further developing results for people encountering a heart attack.

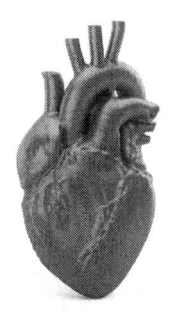

# CHAPTER 5

understanding the reasons for a cardiovascular failure

**1. Atherosclerosis: The Quiet Buildup**

Atherosclerosis is an essential fundamental reason for coronary episodes.

It's a progressive cycle where greasy stores, cholesterol, calcium, and different substances gather in the inward walls of the coronary courses, limiting them over the long haul.

This limiting confines blood stream to the heart muscle, expanding the gamble of coronary episodes.

## 2. High Blood Pressure:

Hypertension (hypertension) is a critical gamble factor for cardiovascular failures.

Uncontrolled hypertension can harm the supply routes, making them more vulnerable to atherosclerosis and plaque development.

It likewise expands the responsibility on the heart, possibly prompting heart muscle thickening and debilitating.

## 3. Cholesterol and Triglycerides

Raised degrees of LDL cholesterol (frequently alluded to as "awful" cholesterol) in the blood can add to atherosclerosis.

At the point when LDL cholesterol joins with different substances, it structures plaque in the courses.

High fatty oil levels, one more sort of blood fat, can likewise be related with an expanded gamble of respiratory failures.

## 4. Diabetes and Insulin Resistance

Diabetes and insulin opposition can altogether raise the gamble of cardiovascular failures.

High glucose levels related with diabetes can harm veins and advance atherosclerosis.

Insulin opposition, where the body's cells don't answer really to insulin, can prompt high glucose and expanded cardiovascular gamble.

# CHAPTER 6

## 1 Anticipation Strategies

Forestalling a coronary failure includes embracing an all encompassing way to deal with heart wellbeing.

Different procedures can essentially decrease the gamble of coronary episodes and advance in general cardiovascular prosperity.

## 2. Diet and Nutrition

A heart-sound eating regimen is urgent in forestalling coronary episodes.

Zero in on:

Eating different foods grown from the ground.

Picking entire grains over refined ones.

Settling on lean proteins like fish, poultry, and vegetables.

Diminishing immersed and trans fats.

Restricting salt admission.

Watching segment sizes.

An even eating regimen can assist with controlling cholesterol levels, circulatory strain, and glucose.

A respiratory failure patient ought to zero in on a heart-sound eating regimen to help recuperation and diminish the gamble of future heart issues. Here are food sources to eat and food sources to stay away from:

**Food varieties to Eat (Heart-Sound Choices)**

1.Fruits and Vegetables:

These are plentiful in nutrients, minerals, fiber, and cell reinforcements. Hold back nothing of brilliant choices like berries, mixed greens, citrus organic products, and carrots.

2. Whole Grains:

Settle on entire grains like oats, earthy colored rice, entire wheat bread, and quinoa. They give fundamental supplements and fiber.

3. Lean Proteins:

Pick lean wellsprings of protein like skinless poultry, fish (particularly greasy fish like salmon and mackerel), vegetables (beans and lentils), and tofu.

4. Healthy Fats:

Incorporate wellsprings of sound fats like avocados, nuts (e.g., almonds, pecans), seeds (e.g., flaxseeds, chia seeds), and olive oil. These fats can assist with bringing down awful cholesterol levels.

5. Low-Fat Dairy:

In the event that you consume dairy items, decide on low-fat or without fat variants to decrease immersed fat admission.

## 6. Fish Oil:

Greasy fish or fish oil enhancements can give omega-3 unsaturated fats, which are helpful for heart wellbeing.

## 7. Nuts:

with some restraint, nuts like almonds and pecans can be a heart-sound nibble because of their unsaturated fats, fiber, and cell reinforcements.

## 8. Legumes:

Beans, lentils, and chickpeas are astounding wellsprings of plant-based protein and fiber.

## 9. Fiber-Rich Foods:

Food sources high in solvent fiber, similar to oats, beans, and natural products, can assist with bringing down cholesterol levels.

## Food varieties to Stay away from (Cutoff or Stay away from These):

1. Saturated and Trans Fats:

Lessen admission of food varieties high in immersed fats, like red meat, full-fat dairy items, and broiled food varieties. Stay away from trans fats tracked down in many handled and broiled food varieties.

2. Added Sugars:

Cutoff sweet beverages, desserts, and handled food varieties that contain added sugars, as extreme sugar admission can add to coronary illness.

3. High-Sodium Foods:

Lessen salt admission by keeping away from high-sodium handled food sources, canned soups, and vigorously salted snacks. Use spices and flavors for flavor rather than salt.

## 4. Processed Meats:

Limit utilization of handled meats like frankfurters, sausages, and bacon, as they are high in soaked fats and sodium.

## 5. Excess Alcohol:

Breaking point liquor utilization to direct levels or as suggested by your medical services supplier. Extreme liquor can adversely affect the heart.

## 6. Fast Food and Broiled Foods:

Keep away from or limit cheap food and seared food varieties because of their high soaked fat and calorie content.

7. Large Meals:
Choose more modest, more regular feasts to forestall gorging and decrease the responsibility on your heart.

8. Trans-Fat-Containing Oils:
Check food names and stay away from items made with to some extent hydrogenated oils, a wellspring of trans fats.

It's fundamental for cardiovascular failure patients to work with an enlisted dietitian or medical services supplier to make a customized eating plan custom-made to their particular requirements and hazard factors. Following a heart-solid eating regimen, joined with way of life changes and medicine the executives, can essentially further develop heart wellbeing and decrease the risk of future cardiovascular occasions.

## 3. Practice and Actual Activity

Customary actual work is fundamental for heart wellbeing.

Go for the gold 150 minutes of moderate-power high-impact practice or 75 minutes of enthusiastic power practice each week.

Exercises like energetic strolling, swimming, or cycling can work on cardiovascular wellness, lower circulatory strain, and diminish the gamble of heftiness.

## 4. Stress Management

Ongoing pressure can add to coronary illness risk.

Methods like contemplation, profound breathing activities, yoga, and care can assist with overseeing pressure.

Satisfactory rest and keeping a sound balance between serious and fun activities are likewise essential for decreasing pressure.

## 5. Drugs and Treatments

Contingent upon individual gamble variables and clinical history, medical services suppliers might prescribe drugs to oversee conditions like hypertension, elevated cholesterol, or diabetes.

Now and again, ibuprofen or other blood-diminishing prescriptions might be endorsed to forestall blood clusters.

Strategies like angioplasty and stent position or coronary course sidestep uniting (CABG) might be important to treat critical blockages in the coronary corridors.

Avoidance is key with regards to cardiovascular failures. By embracing a heart-sound way of life that incorporates a fair eating regimen, normal activity, stress the board, and, when vital, proper clinical medicines, people can fundamentally lessen their gamble of coronary illness and respiratory failures. Talking with a medical care supplier for customized direction is fundamental in making a viable counteraction plan.

## CHAPTER 7

### 1. Medications

Meds assume a basic part in overseeing cardiovascular failures and forestalling further complexities.

Normal prescriptions endorsed during and after a cardiovascular failure include:

**Aspirin**

Frequently given during a respiratory failure to lessen blood clump development.

**Thrombolytic (Cluster Busting) Drugs**

These medications can break down blood clumps that are impeding coronary supply routes.

**Antiplatelet Agents Prescriptions like**

clopidogrel are utilized to forestall future blood clusters.

### Beta-Blockers

These assist with lessening pulse and circulatory strain, alleviating the heart's responsibility.

### ACE Inhibitors or ARBs

These medications are utilized to bring down pulse and decrease stress on the heart.

### Statins

Recommended to bring down cholesterol levels and lessen the gamble of future heart occasions.

## 2. Angioplasty and Stenting

Percutaneous Coronary Intercession (PCI), normally known as angioplasty, is a technique to open obstructed coronary supply routes.

During angioplasty, a catheter with an inflatable is embedded into the restricted vein and swelled to extend it.

Frequently, a stent (a little cross section tube) is set to keep the corridor open.

Angioplasty and stenting are typically performed for both crisis treatment during a cardiovascular failure (essential angioplasty) and as elective methodology for patients with critical blockages.

### 3. Sidestep A medical procedure (Coronary Conduit Sidestep Joining - CABG)

CABG is a surgery used to sidestep hindered or restricted coronary supply routes.

A specialist takes a solid vein from one more piece of the body, generally the chest or leg, and joins it to the coronary conduits to make another course for blood stream.

This medical procedure is commonly saved for cases with different or extreme blockages that can't be successfully treated with angioplasty or meds.

## 4. Cardiovascular Rehabilitation

Cardiovascular restoration is an organized program that assists people with recuperating from a coronary failure or heart medical procedure.

It incorporates observed work out, schooling on heart-solid living, and consistent reassurance.

Cardiovascular recovery can work on actual wellness, decrease the gamble of future heart issues, and upgrade generally speaking prosperity.

The decision of treatment relies upon factors like the seriousness of the coronary episode, the degree of supply route blockages, and the patient's general wellbeing. Treatment plans are frequently custom fitted to individual necessities, and a medical services supplier will examine the most reasonable choices for every patient's particular circumstance.

## What to do when heart attack happens

On the off chance that you or somebody you are with encounters side effects that might demonstrate a coronary failure, it's pivotal to rapidly act. Here are the moves you can take when a cardiovascular failure occurs:

## 1. Call Emergency Services:

Promptly call your nearby Emergency number (e.g., 911 in the US) to demand a rescue vehicle. Time is basic in limiting heart muscle harm during a coronary failure, delay don't as well.

## 2. Take Ibuprofen/Aspirin (If Advised):

In the event that you have been recommended anti-inflamatory medicine by your medical care supplier and it is promptly accessible, and you are not susceptible to it, you can bite and swallow one ordinary (325 mg) headache medicine tablet. Headache medicine can assist with forestalling further blood cluster development.

### 3. Stay Quiet and Rest:
Sit or rests in an agreeable position and attempt to remain as quiet as could really be expected. Keep away from any actual effort, as this can strain your heart further.

### 4. Do Not Drive Yourself:
It's fundamental not to endeavor to head to the medical clinic. Trust that the rescue vehicle will show up, as they are prepared to give quick clinical consideration.

### 5. Loosen Tight Clothing:

In the event that you are wearing tight clothing, like a tie or belt, consider slackening or eliminating it to make breathing simpler.

## 6. Stay Conscious and Alert:

On the off chance that you're separated from everyone else, remain conscious and alert until crisis administrations show up. In the event that you're with somebody who is encountering a cardiovascular failure, console and keep them alert on the off chance that they are cognizant.

Recall that not all heart attack present with serious chest torment. Side effects can change, and a few people might encounter milder inconvenience, windedness, queasiness, or other surprising sensations. In the event that you suspect a respiratory failure or notice somebody giving these indications, decide in favor watchfulness and look for guaranteed clinical consideration. Early mediation can have a massive effect in the result and limit harm to the heart muscle.

## Reversing Heart Attack Requires the following steps:

**1. Consult a Medical services Provider**
Start by counseling a medical care supplier, ideally a cardiologist, to survey your condition, risk variables, and generally speaking heart wellbeing. They can give a customized treatment plan.

**2. Medications**
Your doctor might endorse meds to oversee risk factors, for example, hypertension, elevated cholesterol, or

diabetes. Accepting these prescriptions as coordinated is urgent.

## 3. Lifestyle Changes

Diet

Embrace a heart-sound eating routine wealthy in natural products, vegetables, entire grains, lean proteins (e.g., fish, poultry, vegetables), and low-fat dairy items. Limit immersed and trans fats, sodium, and added sugars.

**Exercise**

Participate in standard active work, going for the gold 150 minutes of moderate-power high-impact practice or 75 minutes of fiery power practice each week. Counsel your medical services supplier prior to beginning another work-out daily practice.

**Smoking Cessation**

Quit smoking in the event that you smoke, as it is a huge gamble factor for coronary illness.

**Weight Management**

Accomplish and keep a sound load through a blend of diet and exercise. Indeed, even unassuming weight reduction can decidedly affect heart wellbeing.

### Stress Management

Practice pressure decrease methods like profound breathing, contemplation, yoga, or care to actually oversee pressure.

### 4. Nutritional Supplements

Examine with your medical care supplier whether enhancements like omega-3 unsaturated fats, coenzyme Q10 (CoQ10), or garlic might be useful for your heart wellbeing.

### 5. Cardiac Rehabilitation

On the off chance that you've had a coronary failure or gone through heart-related methods, consider signing up for a cardiovascular restoration program. These projects give practice preparing, training, and basic encouragement.

### 6. Monitoring

Consistently screen your circulatory strain, cholesterol levels, and glucose in the event that you have diabetes. This helps track progress and guarantees that your drugs and way of life changes are viable.

## 7. Limit Alcohol

Assuming you drink liquor, do as such with some restraint. Exorbitant liquor utilization can add to coronary illness.

## 8. Stay Informed

Teach yourself about heart wellbeing, risk factors, and cautioning signs. Information enables you to settle on informed choices.

## 9. Sleep Well

Go for the gold long stretches of value rest each evening. Unfortunate rest can adversely influence heart wellbeing.

## 10. Social Support

Encircle yourself with steady loved ones who empower and build up your solid way of life decisions.

Recall that reversing coronary illness is a continuous interaction, and results might fluctuate relying upon individual variables. It's fundamental for work intimately with your medical services supplier to create and keep a customized plan custom-made to your necessities. Standard subsequent arrangements are essential to follow headway and make fundamental changes in accordance with your treatment plan.

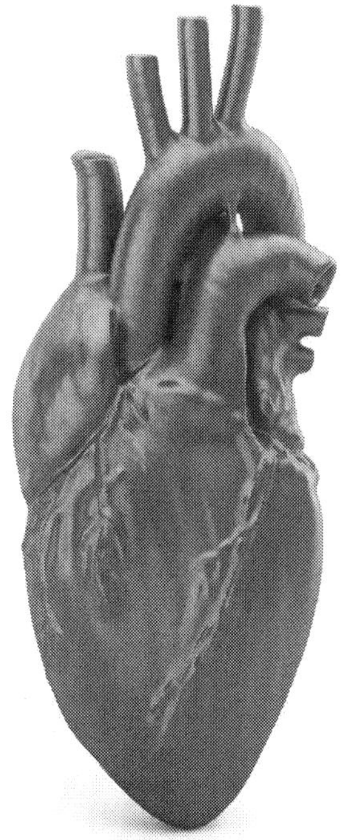

# CHAPTER 8

## LIFE AFTER HEART ATTACK

**1 Adapting to the Aftermath**

Adapting to life after a coronary failure can genuinely challenge.

Normal feelings incorporate tension, dread, and discouragement.

Looking for help from medical care experts, companions, and family can assist with dealing with these sentiments.

**2. Way of life Changes for Recovery**

Recuperation from a coronary failure frequently includes making critical way of life changes to lessen the gamble of future heart issues. Key changes include:

**Dietary Adjustments**

Embracing a heart-solid eating routine low in immersed fats, sodium, and handled food varieties.

**Ordinary Exercise:**

Bit by bit integrating actual work into day to day schedules under clinical direction.

**Smoking Cessation**

Stopping smoking to diminish the gamble of additional heart issues.

**Medicine Adherence**

Reliably taking endorsed prescriptions to oversee pulse, cholesterol, and other gamble factors.

### 3. Profound Well-being

Profound wellbeing is vital to the recuperation cycle.

Meeting with a specialist or instructor can assist with overseeing pressure, uneasiness, or sorrow.

Unwinding strategies and care practices can uphold close to home prosperity.

## 4. Support Systems

The help of loved ones is imperative during recuperation.

Joining support gatherings or taking part in cardiovascular recovery programs associates you with other people who have encountered comparative difficulties.

Sharing encounters and counsel can offer profound and reasonable help.

# HEART ATTACK UNMASKED

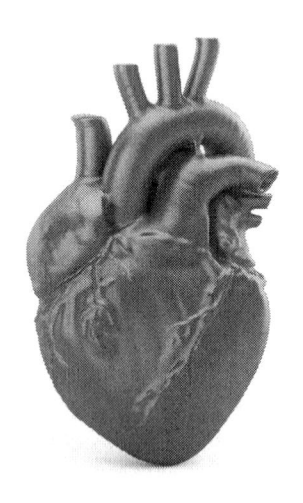

# CHAPTER 9

**1. Mending and Recovery**

Recuperation from a respiratory failure is a progressive interaction that includes mending the heart muscle and tending to fundamental gamble factors.

It's fundamental to follow clinical proposals and stick to way of life changes to advance ideal recuperation.

## 2. Actual Rehabilitation

- Actual recovery might be prescribed to further develop strength, perseverance, and generally speaking actual wellbeing.

- Redone practice programs are intended to address individual issues, bit by bit expanding in power as you progress.

## 3. Heart Restoration Programs

Cardiovascular restoration programs are organized to help people recuperating from coronary failures and other heart-related conditions.

## These projects regularly include:

i: Observed Exercise

Administered actual work to work on cardiovascular wellness while guaranteeing wellbeing.

ii: Education

Useful meetings on heart-sound living, prescription administration, and chance element decrease.

iii: Close to home Support

Direction on overseeing pressure, tension, and melancholy.

iv: Way of life Modification

Techniques for keeping a heart-sound eating regimen and normal active work.

Heart recovery programs are advantageous in upgrading physical and close to home prosperity during recuperation.

## 4. Diet and Exercise Plans

Enlisted dietitians and exercise experts team up to make customized plans for post-coronary episode patients.

**Dietary Plans**

Accentuation on heart-solid nourishment, including expanded admission of organic products, vegetables, entire grains, lean proteins, and decreased utilization of soaked fats and sodium.

Practice Plans

Steady joining of actual work into day to day existence, with an intend to work on cardiovascular wellness and generally speaking wellbeing.

These plans are intended to forestall further heart issues and advance long haul prosperity.

## 5. Checking Your Advancement

Normal subsequent meetings with medical care suppliers are crucial for screen your heart wellbeing progress.

During these visits, circulatory strain, cholesterol levels, and other fundamental pointers are checked to guarantee you are on the correct way.

Acclimations to prescription and way of life proposals might be gained depending on the situation in light of your headway.

Post-cardiovascular failure recuperation is an excursion that requires responsibility and backing. Actual recovery, cooperation in cardiovascular restoration programs, adherence to dietary and exercise plans, and reliable observing of your advancement are key parts in accomplishing a sound and satisfying life after a coronary failure.

It's critical to work intimately with your medical care group and find proactive ways to keep up with your heart wellbeing.

HEART ATTACK UNMASKED

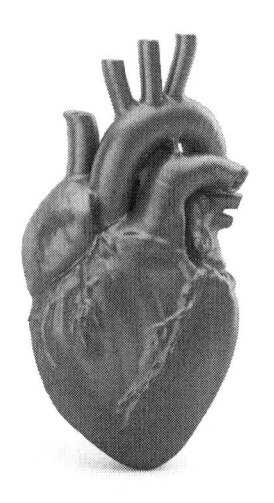

## CONCLUSION

In this excursion through the universe of heart wellbeing, we've explored the unpredictable activities of the human heart, demystified the quiet danger of coronary episodes, and dug into the elements that impact our cardiovascular prosperity. From understanding the reasons for coronary illness to embracing counteraction and treatment procedures, we've strolled the way toward a heart-solid life.

As we are concluding, I need to leave you with a couple of key focal points:

1. Your Heart Matters: Your heart isn't simply an organ; the help supports your whole body. Really focusing on it ought to be a main concern.

2. Knowledge Is Power: Understanding the gamble factors, cautioning signs, and treatment choices for coronary illness engages you to come to informed conclusions about your heart wellbeing.

3. Prevention Is Paramount: Anticipation is the foundation of heart wellbeing. Little, steady changes in your way of life can improve things greatly in safeguarding your heart.

4. Recovery Is Possible: Assuming you've encountered a heart-related occasion, realize that recuperation isn't just imaginable yet in addition reachable. With the right help and responsibility, you can recover your heart's solidarity and flexibility.

5. Support Frameworks Matter: Whether it's the direction of medical services experts, the affection for loved ones, or the fellowship of care groups, your excursion to heart wellbeing isn't one you need to take alone.

6. A Heart-Solid Life Is Worth It: The way to a heart-sound life might be loaded up with difficulties, however the prizes are boundless. Living with reason, defining objectives, and keeping up with heart wellbeing won't just add a very long time to your life yet in addition life to your years.

Recall that your heart is fit for incredible strength and flexibility. It can adjust and mend, and it can keep on beating with reason for a long time to come. By embracing the information and devices gave in this book, you are taking the first and most significant stage toward a heart-solid future.

Your heart deserves the best care, and you have the ability to give it. Let your excursion to heart wellbeing be a demonstration of your obligation to life, love, and every one of the delightful minutes that lie ahead.

Thank you for embarking on this excursion with me. Here's to a heart-solid vital, lovely life loaded up with imperativeness, reason, and vast conceivable outcomes.

Please feel free to leave your review, keep staying healthy, happy heart! ♥, love you.

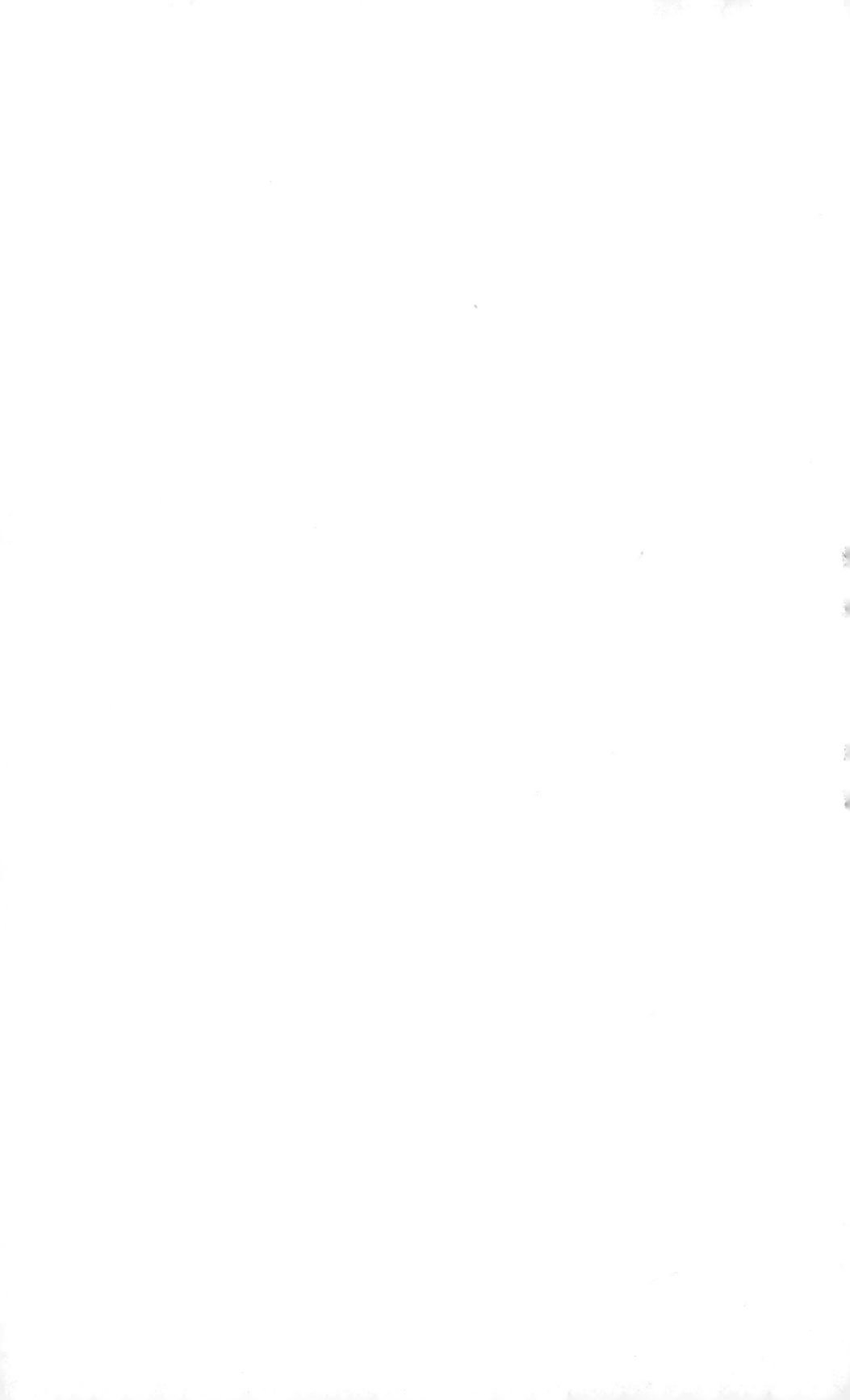

Printed in Great Britain
by Amazon